Victim Advocate's Guide to Wellness:
Six Dimensions of Vicarious Trauma-Free Life

OLGA PHOENIX, MPA, MA

DEDICATION

This book is for all the amazing, beautiful, dedicated, and committed Wonder Women and Wonder Men who create social change daily, participate in elimination of human suffering in the world, and make a difference in the lives of other people on regular basis. You rock my world! And the worlds of many a people who have an honor and a privilege to meet you!

Thank you for being YOU!

CONTENTS

ACKNOWLEDGEMENT

I would like to express my deepest gratitude to vicarious trauma researchers, practitioners, and authors, who influenced and inspired me: Karen Saakvine, Laurie Anne Pearlman, Charles Figley, Beth Stamm, Laura van Dernoot Lypsky, Sandra Bloom, Naomi Rachel Remen, Francoise Mathieu, John Fawcett, and many others.

I would like to thank Pamela Jacobs, a friend and a visionary, from the bottom of my heart, for helping me conceive Olga Phoenix Project: Healing for Social Change, and this book- this all would not be possible without you, my friend! To my birth family-Vitalik, t. Luba, d.Vova, Mama, Busek, d.Vitya, - thank you for all the lessons you taught me, I love you, always. To my chosen family-Annette, Gig, and the kids, Barbara C., Fran, Louise L., Meg P., Laura C. R., Melody T., Jenn M., Kimberly G., Rosa M., Dr. Joan P., Dr. Jane C., Denny M., and many, many brothers and sisters all over the world -thank you for saving my life and loving me until I could love myself. To the people who helped me heal-Barbara Burkhardt, Diane Edmond, Pal Powell, Dr. John Steele-thank you for showing me the truth.

To all the trauma professionals I've had a fortune to work with- I love your courage, your tenacity, your empathy, your kindness, and your desire to make this world a better place! We are creating social change, my friends! One day at a time, one step at a time! May all our paths be blessed.

INTRODUCTION

Between 40%-85% of "helping professionals" develop vicarious trauma, compassion fatigue and high rates of traumatic symptoms (Mathieu, 2012).

How do we become vicarious trauma statistics?

Seven years ago, I was training new domestic violence advocates on the topic of "Domestic Violence and Children Who Witness It." In the middle of my training, I called for an emergency break and asked my training partner to continue without me. I ran outside, nauseated, covered in cold sweat, my heart exploding out of my chest, and ready to pass out. I was experiencing a full

7

blown panic attack as a result of the material I was presenting. Back then, it didn't occur to me to connect my adverse reaction to the fact that I witnessed my father murdering my mother as a child.

After that panic attack incident, my family and friends urged me to leave the field, concerned about my mental and physical health, my nightmares, my growing isolation and withdrawal, and my lack of life outside of work. I stayed because I felt that I had to stay no matter what —for my mom. I felt like I owed her that, to be working towards the prevention of domestic violence.

Seven year ago, I thought that I was a Wonder Woman and my past did not define me. I still think exactly the same, except now I know that to help someone else heal, I first have to heal my own personal wounds, and then continue practicing radical vicarious trauma prevention and wellness to maintain a life free of vicarious trauma while working in the trauma field. The majority of us come to trauma-related work for a reason, often having our personal untreated histories of trauma, which makes us vulnerable to vicarious traumatization.

My supervisor suggested I try therapy. That was one of the best suggestions that I ever took, and it started my seven year journey to healing and wellness. After a while, I learned that I don't owe anything to anyone, including my mom. I do this work because it inspires, empowers, and moves me. I *get* to do this work because I feel like I am contributing to bettering of the world, and that makes me feel like a real Wonder Woman. But in order to get to work in the trauma field, I must take care of myself. I must put myself first, always, because doing this is not selfish, but brave and effective. Putting myself first keeps me healthy and balanced in all areas of my life, for me, for my family, and for my clients.

As victim advocates (helping/trauma professionals) we tend to wrap our whole identity around our work, our partner, and/or our children, trying to please everyone. We are constantly reaching for perfection, and forgetting ourselves in the process. We often fall short of our unreachable expectations. Perfection is impossible. Perfection is really a myth, created to keep us forever dissatisfied, guilty, and ashamed of ourselves. We are always striving for more, better, faster, but keep coming up short. This cycle, which keeps us out of balance, prevents us from building a healthy and full life.

I must foster and nurture life outside of work. I need to know I am not just a "victim advocate." I am a friend, a sister, a mother, a cousin, an auntie. I am a spiritual, vulnerable seeker of wisdom, and an ocean lover. I can be intellectual, connected with nature, goofy, and loud at times. Sometimes I just feel lazy and want to escape to Tahiti. I am also a student, a writer, a world traveler, and a lover, who is full of life and gratitude. I can be a compassionate self-forgiver who is sometimes very hard on myself, but I know that life is a journey, not a destination. It's progress, not perfection that counts. There are a myriad of facets of me, and this doesn't even scratch the surface. I know the same is true for you.

Most of us, victims advocates and other trauma professionals, love our jobs. We are often individuals who want to change the world, to eliminate human suffering, to make a difference in the lives of other people. And in our jobs, we can do it all! We are the Wonder Women and Wonder Men who create social change daily. We are also people who have real troubles with taking care of ourselves, who feel guilty about taking vacations, who only take a break when we are really sick, who expect perfection of ourselves. The results are tragic, really. We lose committed, dedicated, and deeply caring trauma professionals to vicarious trauma, compassion fatigue, and burnout.

Like me, you may have wondered: How do I prevent vicarious trauma, compassion fatigue, and burnout from creeping into my life? How do I do this all as a victim advocate, often overworked, underpaid, emotionally, and physically drained? Fortunately, vicarious trauma is preventable. This book is your personal guide to living healthy and content while thriving in a trauma-related field.

Here, you will discover powerful, real life tools for addressing and transforming vicarious trauma and compassion fatigue. You will learn about effective techniques for self-soothing, renewal, and transformation. You will explore breathing modalities, guided meditations, affirmations, gratitude fostering, and leaving work at work rituals to open a way to compassion satisfaction, personal wellness, and empowerment. You will be provided tools to implement, empower, and practice an organizational culture of sustainability and vicarious trauma prevention. Finally, you will find out how to maintain life balance by nurturing physical, psychological, emotional, spiritual, personal, and professional aspects of yourself, in order to create a productive, full, and cherished life free of vicarious trauma.

CHAPTER 1:

WHAT IS VICARIOUS TRAUMA?

Vicarious trauma, secondary traumatic stress or compassion fatigue, trauma exposure response, and burnout are all forms of stress that may affect those working in "helping" professions, because that work involves direct exposure to other's trauma. In the past twenty years there has been a movement to bring awareness and solutions to the profound negative psychological effects caused by being exposed to the trauma of others – ranging from a serious injury to the body from violence or an accident to an emotional wound creates lasting damage to a person's psyche.

Research indicates that domestic and sexual violence advocates, therapists, nurses, physicians, social workers, law enforcement professionals, prosecutors and judges, an astounding number of people in the "helping" professions, are being affected by vicarious trauma, compassion fatigue, secondary trauma, and burnout (Figley, 1996; Maslach, 1996; Saakvitne & Pearlman, 1996; Baird & Jenkins, 2003; Mathieu, 2012).

Definitions

Vicarious trauma, secondary traumatic stress or compassion fatigue, trauma exposure response, and burnout are all forms of stress that may affect those working with victims of violence because that work involves direct exposure to other's trauma. Let's take a closer look at each of the terms.

Vicarious Trauma

Laurie Anne Pearlman and Karen Saakvitne (1996) coined the term Vicarious Traumatization (VT) to describe the profound shift that workers in helping professions experience as "a result of empathic engagement with survivor clients and their trauma material.'" (p.25). According to Pearlman and Saakvitne, VT is an occupational hazard, and unavoidable effect of trauma work, a "human consequence of knowing, caring, and facing the reality of trauma" (1996, p.25).

Trauma workers offer empathetic connection to trauma survivors, and are often profoundly moved by survivors' past experiences. At the same time, trauma work and recovery are often a slow process with a lot of setbacks. This combination of empathetic engagement with multiple survivors over time, a strong desire to help, and the slow recovery process may translate into a vicarious trauma experience for helping professionals.

The main symptoms of VT involve psychological changes in one's system of beliefs around safety, trust, esteem, intimacy, and control regarding both self and others. These changes may have a negative effect on the helper's feelings, relationships, and personal life as well as work with clients. Painful images and emotions related to the client's traumatic memories may become incorporated into the helper's imagery system of memory. This re-experiencing or avoidance of specific aspects of their client's traumatic memories becomes tangible via flashbacks, dreams, painful emotions, or intrusive thoughts.

Secondary Traumatic Stress/Compassion Fatigue

Charles Figley (1983) defined secondary traumatic stress, which he later called compassion fatigue (Figley, 1995), as the experiencing of emotional duress in persons who have had close contact with a trauma survivor, which may include family members as well as therapists. Secondary traumatic stress disorder (STSD) symptoms include re-experiencing the survivor's traumatic event, avoidance, and/or numbing in response to reminders of this event, and persistent arousal (Figley, 1995).

Compassion fatigue (CF) refers to the emotional and physical exhaustion that helping professionals may develop over the course of their careers. It is a gradual negative transformation of helpers' outlook on life: becoming dispirited, bitter, contributing to a toxic work environment, becoming avoidant of clients and family, and experiencing a growing belief in the ineffectiveness of one's work (Mathieu, 2012). Ironically, helpers who are worn out, traumatized, and fatigued, often tend to work harder, thus going further down a dangerous path, which often leads to physical and mental health difficulties, such as depression, chronic pain, substance abuse, and even suicide (Mathieu, 2012, p.9).

Trauma Exposure Response

Laura van Dernoot Lypsky (2009) proposed a new term, trauma exposure response, which she defines as "transformation that takes place within us as a result of exposure to the suffering of other living beings on the planet. This transformation can result from deliberate or inadvertent exposure, formal or informal contact, paid or volunteer work...We are talking about ways in which the world looks and feel like a different place to you as a result of doing your work"(p.41). She describes her experiences with trauma exposure that accumulated while working with survivors of sexual and domestic violence. "I finally came to understand that my exposure to other people's trauma had changed me on a fundamental level," van Dernoot Lypsky writes. "There had been an osmosis: I had absorbed and accumulated trauma to the point that it had become part of me, and my world view has changed" (p.3).

Burnout

Generally speaking, burnout is a term used to describe physical and emotional exhaustion caused by low job satisfaction and feelings of powerlessness and/or inability to change either the work environment or the lives of one's clients. Beth Stamm describes burnout as "the chronicity, acuity and complexity that is perceived to be beyond the capacity of the service provider (Figley, 1995, p.12). Burnout may affect helping professionals in addition to compassion fatigue, but burnout does not mean the negative transformation of one's worldview due to traumatic content of one's clients. Burnout affects people in non-helping professions as well due to having poor pay, unrealistic demands, heavy workload, heavy shifts, poor management, and inadequate supervision, and can happen in any occupation (Mathieu, 2012 p.14).

What's the difference in the terms?

The terms "compassion fatigue," "vicarious traumatization," "secondary traumatization," and "burnout" are used in the literature, sometimes interchangeably and sometimes as distinct constructs. As stated previously in the terminology portion of the section, the term "vicarious trauma" refers to profound negative changes in trauma workers' worldview due to their exposure to traumatic material of their clients; this term will be used throughout this book, although the studies cited may use other terms.

Risk Factors

Clinical and research literature describes a multitude of personal and organizational risk factors associated with vicarious trauma in the victim advocacy field. We cannot change some of them, for instance, a personal history of trauma, but we can definitely modify others, such as learning more positive coping mechanisms or providing vicarious trauma prevention trainings in our agency (Newall &MacNeil, 2010; Bober & Regehr, 2006).

Personal Risk Factors:

- A personal history of trauma
- Preexisting mood disorders
- Unhealthy coping mechanisms
- Being younger in age
- Lack of life outside of work

- Lack of hobbies and support groups
- Having limited professional experience

Organizational Risk Factors:

- Limited supervision
- Working with too many clients
- Geographical and social isolation
- Having limited training about vicarious trauma and its prevention
- Working with a high percentage of traumatized children
- Working with clients who are underserved and disadvantaged
- Working for poor pay, under stressful conditions, with limited resources
- Lack of acknowledgement by agency that vicarious trauma exists

- Lack of acknowledgement by agency that vicarious trauma is a normal reaction to clients' trauma

Warning Signs and Symptoms

Awareness and understanding of warning signs and symptoms of vicarious trauma is of vital importance to its prevention. The symptoms may show up differently in each of us, and knowing how to spot the onset of vicarious trauma can help us to catch it just in time, and start our own preventative measures (Mathieu, 2012; Saakvitne and Pearlman, 1996). The following are symptoms of the onset of vicarious trauma:

Physical: Exhaustion, insomnia, hypersomnia, headaches, and susceptibility to illness.

Behavioral: Increased use of drugs and alcohol, compulsive overeating, other addictions, absenteeism, anger, avoidance of clients, blurred boundaries at work, and isolation.

Psychological: Distancing, negative self-image, depression, inability to empathize, cynicism, bitterness, low job satisfaction and performance, heightened anxiety, irrational fear, problems with intimacy, hypervigilance, intrusive imagery, loss of hope, and the inability to have life outside of work.

Statistics from the Field

Statistics from the field are very consistent: victim advocates suffer "high" to "very high" levels of vicarious trauma, secondary traumatic stress, and compassion fatigue.

Social Workers, MSW:

- 70% exhibited at least one symptom of secondary traumatic stress (Bride, 2007).

Social Workers:

- 42% said they suffered from secondary traumatic stress (Adams et al., 2006).

Social Workers, Domestic Violence and Sexual Assault:

- 65% had at least one symptom of secondary traumatic stress (Bride, 2007).

Forensic Investigators, Internet Crimes Against Children:

- 36% of investigators were experiencing moderate to high levels of secondary trauma (Perez et al., 2010).

Child Welfare Workers:

- 50% of traumatic stress symptoms in severe range (Conrad & Kellar-Guenther, 2006).

Child Welfare Workers:

- 34% met the PTSD diagnostic criteria, due to secondary traumatic stress (Bride, 2007).

Child Protection Service Workers:

- 37% reported clinical levels of emotional distress associated with secondary traumatic stress (Cornille & Meyers, 1999).

Child Protection Workers:

- 50% suffered from "high" to "very high" levels of compassion fatigue (Conrad & Kellar-Guenther, 2006).

Female Forensic Interviewers:

- 34% reported experiencing symptoms of secondary traumatic stress (Perron & Hiltz, 2006).

ProQOL:

Profesional Quality of Life Self-Test

Beth Stamm and Charles Figley have developed a self-test called the ProQOL: Professional Quality of Life Self-Test. The ProQOL is a free tool to assess one's levels of compassion fatigue, burnout and compassion satisfaction.

This test has 30 questions, with five-point scale ranges from never (1) to very often (5), with sub-scales for compassion satisfaction, burnout, and compassion fatigue. This measure has been in use since 1995, and had several revisions, with the latest and most current version called the ProQOL 5 unveiled in 2012. What distinguishes this test from other measures is the notion that helper's professional quality of life is comprised of both positive (compassion satisfaction) and negative (compassion fatigue and burnout) aspects.

Beth Stamm (2010) defines compassion satisfaction as the enjoyment and gratification that professional trauma workers feel when they are able to perform their work well. Helpers who experience compassion satisfaction feel that they are able to handle new responsibilities and want to continue to engage in their work. They feel satisfied and invigorated by the act of helping itself, and by their ability to make constructive difference in their work environment or the larger community. Compassion satisfaction can be fostered by supportive and healthy work environments, self-care, and finding meaning outside of one's work.

I invite you take a few minutes and go over the ProQOL 5 test now. It's reproduced with permissions below in Figure 1. If you would like to download this test online, go to www.proqol.org/ProQol_Test.html.

Beth Stamm encourages everyone who takes this test to submit the results to her, as she is working with this data to study the effectiveness of the test. Please visit her website for more information: www.proqol.org.

Figure 1. Beth Hudnall Stamm, 2009-2012. Professional Quality of Life: Compassion Satisfaction and Fatigue Version 5 (ProQOL). www.proqol.org. Reproduced with permissions.

OLGA PHOENIX

COMPASSION SATISFACTION AND COMPASSION FATIGUE
(PROQOL) VERSION 5 (2009)

When you *[help]* people you have direct contact with their lives. As you may have found, your compassion for those you *[help]* can affect you in positive and negative ways. Below are some questions about your experiences, both positive and negative, as a *[helper]*. Consider each of the following questions about you and your current work situation. Select the number that honestly reflects how frequently you experienced these things in the *last 30 days*.

1=Never	2=Rarely	3=Sometimes	4=Often	5=Very Often

_____ 1. I am happy.

_____ 2. I am preoccupied with more than one person I *[help]*.

_____ 3. I get satisfaction from being able to *[help]* people.

_____ 4. I feel connected to others.

_____ 5. I jump or am startled by unexpected sounds.

_____ 6. I feel invigorated after working with those I *[help]*.

_____ 7. I find it difficult to separate my personal life from my life as a *[helper]*.

_____ 8. I am not as productive at work because I am losing sleep over traumatic experiences of a person I *[help]*.

_____ 9. I think that I might have been affected by the traumatic stress of those I *[help]*.

_____ 10. I feel trapped by my job as a *[helper]*.

_____ 11. Because of my *[helping]*, I have felt "on edge" about various things.

_____ 12. I like my work as a *[helper]*.

_____ 13. I feel depressed because of the traumatic experiences of the people I *[help]*.

_____ 14. I feel as though I am experiencing the trauma of someone I have *[helped]*.

_____ 15. I have beliefs that sustain me.

_____ 16. I am pleased with how I am able to keep up with *[helping]* techniques and protocols.

_____ 17. I am the person I always wanted to be.

_____ 18. My work makes me feel satisfied.

_____ 19. I feel worn out because of my work as a *[helper]*.

_____ 20. I have happy thoughts and feelings about those I *[help]* and how I could help them.

_____ 21. I feel overwhelmed because my case [work] load seems endless.

_____ 22. I believe I can make a difference through my work.

_____ 23. I avoid certain activities or situations because they remind me of frightening experiences of the people I *[help]*.

_____ 24. I am proud of what I can do to *[help]*.

_____ 25. As a result of my *[helping]*, I have intrusive, frightening thoughts.

_____ 26. I feel "bogged down" by the system.

_____ 27. I have thoughts that I am a "success" as a *[helper]*.

_____ 28. I can't recall important parts of my work with trauma victims.

_____ 29. I am a very caring person.

_____ 30. I am happy that I chose to do this work.

Based on your responses, place your personal scores below. If you have any concerns, you should discuss them with a physical or mental health care professional.

Compassion Satisfaction _____

Compassion satisfaction is about the pleasure you derive from being able to do your work well. For example, you may feel like it is a pleasure to help others through your work. You may feel positively about your colleagues or your ability to contribute to the work setting or even the greater good of society. Higher scores on this scale represent a greater satisfaction related to your ability to be an effective caregiver in your job.

The average score is 50 (SD 10; alpha scale reliability .88). About 25% of people score higher than 57 and about 25% of people score below 43. If you are in the higher range, you probably derive a good deal of professional satisfaction from your position. If your scores are below 40, you may either find problems with your job, or there may be some other reason—for example, you might derive your satisfaction from activities other than your job.

Burnout _____

Most people have an intuitive idea of what burnout is. From the research perspective, burnout is one of the elements of Compassion Fatigue (CF). It is associated with feelings of hopelessness and difficulties in dealing with work or in doing your job effectively. These negative feelings usually have a gradual onset. They can reflect the feeling that your efforts make no difference, or they can be associated with a very high workload or a non-supportive work environment. Higher scores on this scale mean that you are at higher risk for burnout.

The average score on the burnout scale is 50 (SD 10; alpha scale reliability .75). About 25% of people score above 57 and about 25% of people score below 43. If your score is below 43, this probably reflects positive feelings about your ability to be effective in your work. If you score above 57 you may wish to think about what at work makes you feel like you are not effective in your position. Your score may reflect your mood; perhaps you were having a "bad day" or are in need of some time off. If the high score persists or if it is reflective of other worries, it may be a cause for concern.

Secondary Traumatic Stress _____

The second component of Compassion Fatigue (CF) is secondary traumatic stress (STS). It is about your work related, secondary exposure to extremely or traumatically stressful events. Developing problems due to exposure to other's trauma is somewhat rare but does happen to many people who care for those who have experienced extremely or traumatically stressful events. For example, you may repeatedly hear stories about the traumatic things that happen to other people, commonly called Vicarious Traumatization. If your work puts you directly in the path of danger, for example, field work in a war or area of civil violence, this is not secondary exposure; your exposure is primary. However, if you are exposed to others' traumatic events as a result of your work, for example, as a therapist or an emergency worker, this is secondary exposure. The symptoms of STS are usually rapid in onset and associated with a particular event. They may include being afraid, having difficulty sleeping, having images of the upsetting event pop into your mind, or avoiding things that remind you of the event.

The average score on this scale is 50 (SD 10; alpha scale reliability .81). About 25% of people score below 43 and about 25% of people score above 57. If your score is above 57, you may want to take some time to think about what at work may be frightening to you or if there is some other reason for the elevated score. While higher scores do not mean that you do have a problem, they are an indication that you may want to examine how you feel about your work and your work environment. You may wish to discuss this with your supervisor, a colleague, or a health care professional.

In this section, you will score your test so you understand the interpretation for you. To find your score on **each section**, total the questions listed on the left and then find your score in the table on the right of the section.

Compassion Satisfaction Scale

Copy your rating on each of these questions on to this table and add them up. When you have added then up you can find your score on the table to the right.

3. _____
6. _____
12. _____
16. _____
18. _____
20. _____
22. _____
24. _____
27. _____
30. _____

Total: _____

The sum of my Compassion Satisfaction questions is	So My Score Equals	And my Compassion Satisfaction level is
22 or less	43 or less	Low
Between 23 and 41	Around 50	Average
42 or more	57 or more	High

Burnout Scale

On the burnout scale you will need to take an extra step. Starred items are "reverse scored." If you scored the item 1, write a 5 beside it. The reason we ask you to reverse the scores is because scientifically the measure works better when these questions are asked in a positive way though they can tell us more about their negative form. For example, question 1. "I am happy" tells us more about

You Wrote	Change to
	5
2	4
3	3
4	2
5	1

the effects of helping when you are not happy so you reverse the score

*1. _____ = _____
*4. _____ = _____
8. _____
10. _____
*15. _____ = _____
*17. _____ = _____
19. _____
21. _____
26. _____
*29. _____ = _____

Total: _____

The sum of my Burnout Questions is	So my score equals	And my Burnout level is
22 or less	43 or less	Low
Between 23 and 41	Around 50	Average
42 or more	57 or more	High

Secondary Traumatic Stress Scale

Just like you did on Compassion Satisfaction, copy your rating on each of these questions on to this table and add them up. When you have added then up you can find your score on the table to the right.

2. _____
5. _____
7. _____
9. _____
11. _____
13. _____
14. _____
23. _____
25. _____
28. _____

Total: _____

The sum of my Secondary Trauma questions is	So My Score Equals	And my Secondary Traumatic Stress level is
22 or less	43 or less	Low
Between 23 and 41	Around 50	Average
42 or more	57 or more	High

CHAPTER 2:

SIX DIMENSIONS OF VT-FREE LIFE

As we have seen, research indicates that continuous exposure to the trauma of others may lead trauma professionals to manifest the same or similar symptoms as the victims they work with. In other words, the symptoms of vicarious trauma (VT) are essentially the same as symptoms of primary trauma, and include re-experience, avoidance, and hyper-arousal. Untreated, VT leads to burnout or compassion fatigue, which manifests in feeling exhausted and worn out; leads to a deep sense of ineffectiveness at one's work; and can result in emotional distress, detachment, ineffective professional behavior, and depression.

Most trauma professionals are aware that vicarious trauma exists, but many may be in denial or have a hard time recognizing VT's impact in their own lives. Laura Van Dernoot Lypsky, a longtime advocate in the field of interpersonal violence prevention, writes about her own difficulty recognizing the negative effects of vicarious trauma in her life, despite repeated encouragement from loved ones to take time off or possibly consider a different line of work. (Lypsky, 2009). She didn't listen for years. Finally, the moment of truth came to her amid her family and friends, while she was on a cliff with a beautiful view. Instead of enjoying her company and the Caribbean Sea, she was thinking about how many people may have killed themselves by jumping off the cliff, and where the nearest trauma center might be. She realized that "she came into work armed with a burning passion and tremendous commitment, but few other internal resources."

Saakvine, Pearlman, Lypsky, and other VT researchers have also exposed the truth about trauma work. Rather than pathologizing the negative effects of working with the trauma of others, they normalize them as natural and universal reactions to trauma, similar to the approaches that trauma professionals take when working with trauma survivors. But more importantly, they offer creative, preventative solutions.

Karen Saakvine and Laurie Anne Pearlman suggest that VT prevention is two-fold: first, we must address the stress of VT through self-care, nurturing activities, and escape. Secondly, we can transform the despair, demoralization, and loss of hope of VT by creating meaning, challenging negative beliefs and assumptions, and participating in community-building activities "While we believe that the effects of vicarious traumatization are inevitable and permanent, we also believe they are modifiable. Thus, while this will change you, there is a lot you can do about it"(Saakvine and Pearlman, 1996). For visual learner, like myself, I've created a graphic of these concepts which you can see in Figure 2.

Figure 2. Vicarious Trauma Prevention is 2-Fold.

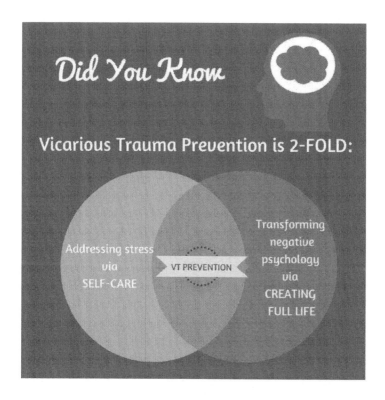

This two-part solution to vicarious trauma is very important. In the past several years self-care in victim advocacy has been brought to the forefront of the movement, and this is great. However, the second part of the solution, the negative psychological effects transforming activities, such as rich life outside of work; identifying, working on, and fulfilling long-term goals; discovering and pursuing your passions; building strong support systems outside of work are not emphasized at all, and often are completely forgotten. Realistically, one cannot transform despair, loss of hope, and nihilism brought on by vicarious trauma by taking a bubble bath or getting a massage. This is just not going to happen. Therefore, when we only talk about self-care as a vicarious trauma prevention tool, we are only talking about half of the solution. And of course, when it comes to vicarious trauma, half measures are very much inadequate.

I have developed a tool designed to help us, as victim advocates, to develop a personal comprehensive vicarious trauma prevention plan that encompasses both self-care activities and vicarious trauma transforming activities, in order to bring wellness, contentment, and joy into our lives. It's called the Life Balance Wheel. Take a look at it in Figure 3. You can download a Life Balance Wheel file in color and bigger size at www.olgaphoenix.com.

Figure 3. Life Balance Wheel.

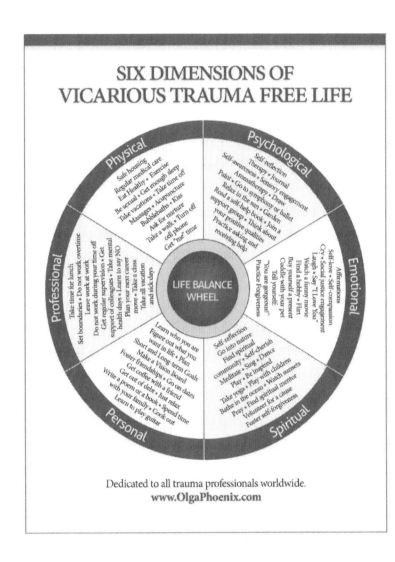

The Life Balance Wheel is designed to help trauma workers live full, vicarious trauma-free lives. The Life Balance Wheel is an empowering, affirming, and positive tool for victim advocates. The Wheel is comprised of six dimensions: physical, psychological, emotional, spiritual, personal, and professional. Each dimension represents a part of our lives which requires our daily attention.

All six dimensions are equally important: without nurturing and addressing our physical needs, we cannot be effective in our professional lives; without cultivating the physiological and emotional aspects of ourselves, we cannot effectively negate the despair, demoralization, and loss of hope imposed by vicarious trauma.

I like to think about the Life Balance Wheel as a bottom of a chair, with its six dimensions being its six legs. My Life Balance chair is steady and supports me perfectly when I nurture and take care of all six dimensions of my life equally. When, however, my focus on certain parts of my life decreases—if, for example, I forget to take care of physical or emotional needs by working too much—my Life Balance chair becomes wobbly and shaky, just the way my life becomes unbalanced and unhealthy. This is when I become especially vulnerable to vicarious trauma and burnout.

In order for the Life Balance Wheel to work, it needs to be preventative and sustainable. It means that we cannot put a copy of the Wheel on our wall at work and expect to never experience the effects of vicarious trauma. The Life Balance Wheel, rather, needs to become an integral part of our life. I invite you to experiment with the 88 suggested exercises on the Life Balance Wheel until you know which ones you want to adapt in your life and then practice it as often as you can.

First, these activities should be done regularly, before a crisis. Say you like a particular guided relaxation meditation on CD. For this meditation to work well for you in a crisis, you must practice it regularly and know for sure it works for you. As the word "preventative" implies, this particular method may prevent you from having to be in a state of crisis in the first place.

Secondly, your vicarious trauma-free lifestyle needs to be sustainable. It means realistic, ongoing efforts which will keep you healthy continuously through your career. For example, I will never become an early bird, thus I know that making myself wake up at 4 am to go to the gym probably will not work in the long run. This type of unrealistic thinking is not only unsustainable, but self-sabotaging. If you pick something you enjoy, it will be so much easier to make it a preventative and sustainable part of your vicarious trauma-free lifestyle.

Life Balance Wheel and Alternative Healing Modalities

Overall, the Life Balance Wheel contains 88 suggestions for a range of vicarious trauma prevention practices, ranging from meeting basic physical needs to finding life's purpose and meaning through the psychological and spiritual dimensions. The goal is to give trauma professionals a great variety of self-care tools so they can explore, test, and adapt them into a personalized, preventative and sustainable vicarious trauma-free lifestyle.

Many of the practices offered in the Life Balance Wheel are recognized as Alternative Healing Modalities. The term Alternative Healing Modalities means any form of treatment that is outside of the mainstream Western medicine. Generally speaking, the Alternative Healing Modalities Model views a human being as a complex organism in which body, mind, and spirit are dynamically interconnected. Mindful, intentional connection between body and mind can have a profound effect on healing. Mood, attitude, and personal beliefs can influence a person's emotional, mental, and physical health. Alternative healing modalities are designed to enhance the mind's positive impact on the body through simple methods, such as mindfulness, meditation, mindful breathing, and various relaxation techniques.

For example, meditation has been used for thousands of years to facilitate healing and alleviate suffering. The calming effects of meditation allow the brain and body to work together more effectively, resulting in clarity of thought, lower blood pressure, and a calmer nervous system. Meditation is widely used to treat mood disorders, high cholesterol, high blood pressure, and headaches. Mary Beth Jansenn (2009), the author of Pleasure Healing: Mindful Practices and Sacred Spa Ritual, reports the following tremendous advantages of meditation:

Meditation can:

- help us develop a thicker cerebral cortex than non-meditators, which means higher levels of mental sharpness;
- promote the rewiring of brain circuitry to make us more resilient;

- create happiness by significantly shifting brain waves from right-prefrontal cortex to left-prefrontal cortex where positive emotions and optimism reside;

- regulate hormones and increase levels of serotonin, the brain feel-good chemical; and

- provide relief from anxiety and depression by lowering levels of cortisol.

There are hundreds of different alternative healing modalities practiced all over the world. The most popular forms of alternative healing modalities practiced in the United States are Acupuncture, Aromatherapy, Art Therapy, Chiropractic, Dance Therapy, Deep Breathing, Herbalism, Guided Imagery, Massage, Meditation, Progressive Muscle Relaxation, Tai Chi, Reiki, Reflexology, and Yoga. Each practice can be easily incorporated in your daily life, providing balance, positive focus, and reprieve when needed. More information about each modality follows:

Acupuncture:

Fine needles are inserted at specific points to stimulate, disperse, and regulate the flow of vital energy, and restore a healthy energy balance.

Aromatherapy:

Using essential oils extracted from plants, aromatherapy treats stress and anxiety. Oils are massaged into the skin in diluted form, inhaled, or placed in baths.

Art Therapy:

Sometimes called creative arts therapy or expressive arts therapy, this type of therapy encourages people to express and understand emotions through artistic expression and through the creative process.

Chiropractic:

The chiropractic care views the misalignments of the vertebrae which cause pressure on the spinal nerve roots, as the root of many illness. The healing is reached by manipulating the vertebrae and releasing spinal pressure.

Dance Therapy:

Dance and/or movement therapy uses expressive movement as a therapeutic tool for both personal expression and psychological or emotional healing.

Deep-breathing:

A simple, yet powerful, relaxation technique and is the cornerstone of many other relaxation practices, and can be combined with other relaxing elements such as aromatherapy and music.

Herbalism:

Herbalism uses natural plants to treat a range of illnesses and to enhance the functioning of the body's systems.

Guided imagery:

Guided imagery is a program of directed thoughts and suggestions that guide one's imagination toward a relaxed, focused state. One can use an instructor, tapes, or scripts to help through this process.

Massage:

General term for a range of therapeutic approaches which involve the practice of manipulating a person's muscles and other soft tissue with the intent of improving a person's well-being.

Meditation:

Private devotion or mental exercise, in which techniques of concentration and contemplation are used to reach a heightened level of spiritual awareness and/or improve a person's well-being.

Progressive muscle relaxation:

Progressive muscle relaxation involves a two-step process in which a person systematically tenses and relaxes different muscle groups in the body. Helps one to spot and counteract the first signs of the muscular tension that accompanies stress.

Tai Chi:

Originally developed for self-defense, Tai Chi has evolved into a graceful form of exercise that's now used for stress reduction and a variety of other health conditions. Often described as meditation in motion, Tai Chi promotes serenity through gentle movements.

Reflexology:

This modality is based on the idea that specific points on the feet and hands correspond with organs and tissues throughout the body. With fingers and thumbs, the practitioner applies pressure to these points to treat a wide range of stress-related illnesses.

Reiki:

Practitioners of this ancient Tibetan healing system use light hand placements to channel healing energies to the recipient, and to assist the recipient in achieving spiritual focus and clarity.

Yoga:

A physical and mental discipline practiced to

attain the physical and emotional balance, achieved through a series of postures and breathing exercises.

CHAPTER 3:

SIX DIMENSIONS IN ACTION

In this chapter, we will explore and practice various exercises from the six dimensions of The Life Balance Wheel. As I said in the previous chapter, the wheel contains 88 various vicarious trauma prevention activities. In this chapter I would like to invite you to practice these activities with me, and see what fits for you. The goal is to pick out one or two activities in each dimension and practice them often, dedicating equal attention to all six dimensions, as they are equally important. If some activity does not work for you, no problem, go back to the Life Balance Wheel and pick something you are interested in, or better yet, put down your own activity that you know will work for you. Eventually, you will have a great range of tools to work with: this will become your trusted Life Balance Plan, encompassing vicarious trauma prevention activities from taking care of body to creating a meaningful life outside of your work. Let's create a preventative, sustainable Life Balance Plan that works for YOU.

1. Physical Dimension

In Crisis? Self-soothe with Your Senses!

First of all, just breathe! Take a giant freeing breath in and out, in and out. Breathe with your belly, in and out, in and out. Relax your shoulders, in and out, in and out. Light-headed yet?

According to the branches of psychology called self-psychology and attachment theory, the ability to regulate our feelings and strong emotions (self-soothing) is at the core of our well-being. Attachment theory suggests we learn self-soothing techniques from our primary caregivers, like parents or guardians. Some of my friends are just natural self-soothers; it's like they went to a special self-soothing class (which I personally missed) in elementary school. Chances are, their parents had strong skills in regulating emotions and they passed it on to their children. Sometimes, we grow up and realize that our primary caregivers gave us only unhealthy coping mechanisms, and then we go to therapy to learn the new positive ways to cope.

In trauma work we are faced with extreme levels of human suffering, and at times our personal and professional crises may trigger a flood of emotions or even produce a dissociative experience. Self-soothing techniques may be life savers as we ride out painful emotions, wait for crisis to pass, and tolerate the feelings of anger, despair, or shame without becoming (self) destructive. There are a thousand and one ways to self-soothe, and each one of us has to stock his or her own self-toolkit with resources that work for them personally. Sometimes, strong feelings and emotions may cause us to completely forget how to self-soothe in a positive manner. I keep an index card in my wallet with my personal self-soothing instructions. This way, if I am very distressed, I can always count on my list to be available at my fingertips.

Using Your Senses to Self-Soothe

I find "Self-soothing with Your 5 Senses" exercises very easy to remember. There are a number of them out there; I will touch upon two that work for me. Generally speaking, when distressed, focus on your senses to clear your mind of negative thoughts. Then, try one of these techniques:

Count of Your Senses 1-2-3-4-5 Technique (Alberts, 2009)

1. State 1 scent you can smell.
2. Name 2 sounds you can hear.
3. Describe 3 sensations your body is feeling.

4. Identify 4 colors you can see.

5. Name 5 things you see in front of you.

Self-soothing with Your 5 Senses Technique (Dialectical Behavior Therapy Skills)

This technique is widely used in Dialectical Behavior Therapy (DBT) for emotional regulation and distress tolerance. Dialectical behavior therapy (DBT) is a form of psychotherapy that was originally developed by Marsha M. Linehan, a psychology researcher at the University of Washington, and author of the *Skills Training Manual for Treating Borderline Personality Disorder,* to treat people with borderline personality disorder (BPD) and chronic suicidality. More recently, researchers like Decker and Naugle have described its use in treating traumatic brain injuries (TBI), post-traumatic stress disorder (PTSD), eating disorders, chemical dependency, sexual abuse, and various mood disorders. DBT patients generally attend group therapy and individual therapy once a week for about a year, where they learn about emotional regulation, distress tolerance, interpersonal effectiveness, acceptance, and mindful awareness, largely based on Buddhist meditative practice.

Here I have included the "Self-soothing with Your 5 Senses" Graphic for you. You can easily make one for yourself with activities that work for you. With practice, you will start to notice that self-soothing in a positive manner comes naturally!

Figure 4. Self-soothe with Five Senses.

CRISIS SURVIVAL SKILLS

Self-Soothe with Five Senses

VISION:
Watch the beauty of nature, look at beautiful photos, art, architecture

TASTE:
Drink chamomile and peppermint tea, eat slowly and mindfully, savoring every bite

HEARING:
Listen to rain, music, birds, ocean waves, children laughing, guided meditation

TOUCH:
Take a bubble bath put clean sheets on your bed, slowly and mindfully pet your animals.

SMELL:
Use your favorite perfume, scented candles, burn sage, cook food, buy flowers

Based on DBT Therapy Skills

≡ WHAT WORKS FOR YOU? ≡

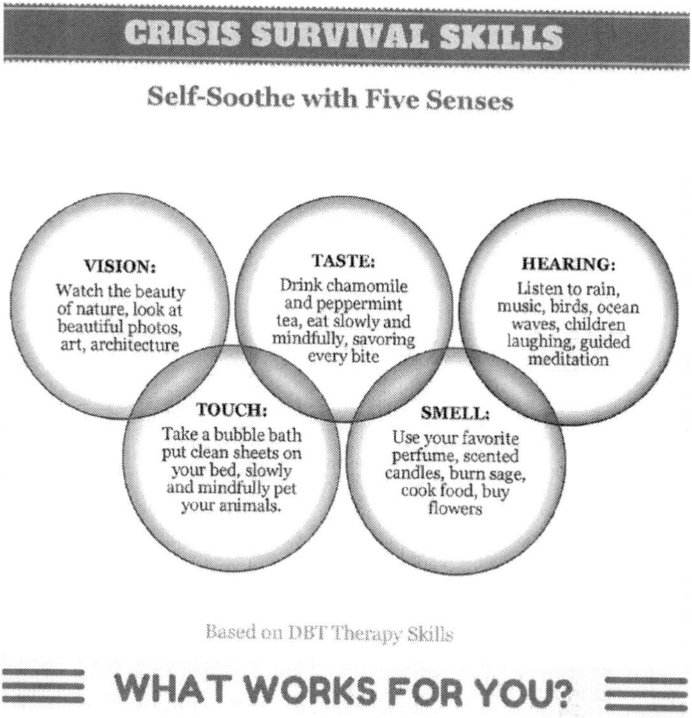

"My Safe Place" 5 Senses Guided Imagery Exercise

When you need immediate stress reduction, My Safe Place 5 Senses Guided Imagery exercise is very effective. The goal of this imagery exercise is to determine your personal safe place, where you can "retreat" to in your mind, self-soothe, and survive a crisis situation without being overwhelmed by negative emotions or being self-destructive. You can practice it with a friend or record it yourself and listen to it when needed. As with all the tools presented in this book, in order to be effective, a particular tool must become a part of your daily self-care and wellness plan. In other words, practice, practice, practice is the key to prevention and sustainability.

Before starting your guided imagery exercise, think of a real or imaginary place which makes you feel safe. For me, sounds and images of the ocean are always the way to go. Others prefer mountains, cabins by the sea, infinite fields of flowers, or simply sitting on a big cloud in the sky, feeling safe. For inspiration, take a look at some of my personal favorites, in Figure 5. Choose your place and then you can begin the guided imagery.

Figure 5. Safe Place Guided Imagery

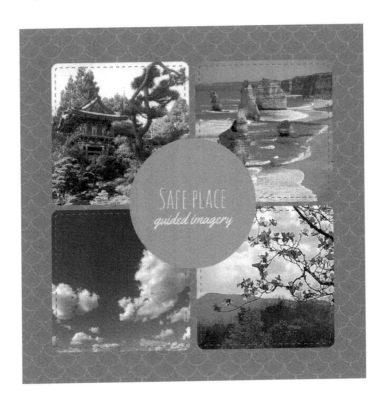

Instructions:

To begin, sit in a comfortable position with your back straight, your feet flat on the floor, and your hands placed comfortably in your lap. You may close your eyes if you wish. Start by breathing in and out, in and out, feeling the calm and relaxation slowly entering your body. Feel your belly expand like a balloon, in and out. Continue breathing deeply and slowly for the rest of the exercise.

Now imagine your safe place using all your five senses in order to really ground yourself in the scene.

Vision: What do you see? What does this place look like? Is it indoors or out? Is it day or night? Do you see the sun, moon, stars, rain, or snow? Do you see other people or animals? Take a few moments breathing deeply and looking around your safe place.

Hearing: What do you hear? Birds, animals, music, waves, silence? Choose a soothing sound and concentrate on it for a few moments, breathing in and out, in and out.

Smell: What do you smell? Ocean, rain, storm, fireplace, dinner cooking, flowers, breeze, your pets? Pick a soothing smell and concentrate on it for a few moments, breathing deeply in and out, in and out.

Touch: What can you touch in your imaginary safe place? Sand, water, fur, velvet fabric, fresh cut grass? Choose something soothing to touch for a few moments, breathing deeply in and out, in and out.

Taste: Is there something you can taste in your imaginary safe place? Chamomile tea, watermelon, ocean spray, dinner? Concentrate on something soothing to taste and breathe deeply for a few moments.

Now take a few moments to explore your imaginary safe place with all of your senses. Think about how safe, soothed, and relaxed you feel here. Make a mental note for yourself that you can come back here any time you need to feel safe and relaxed. You can come back when you are in crisis, had a bad day, or just want to get away and breathe deeply for a while.

Continue breathing deeply, in and out, in and out. Feel your body being relaxed and safe. When you are ready, open your eyes and come to your usual level of wakefulness and alertness. You are safe, soothed, and relaxed. Everything will be alright.

2. Psychological Dimension

With a good grounding in our physical bodies, we can go on to address psychological pathways to healing. Sometimes changing your psychological mindset is as easy as letting go of the one negative element that's getting you down and focusing instead on the dozens of positives.

Our Negativity Bias

Dr. Rick Hanson introduced ground-breaking research in his book *Just One Thing*. In it, he writes that scientists believe that our human brain has a built-in negativity bias. This is because, as our ancestors struggled for survival over millions of years of evolution, negative thinking—such as fear and being alert to potential dangers—had a greater impact on survival than positive thinking, which might lead someone to dismiss real dangers. The brain generally reacts more strongly to a negative stimulus than to an equally intense positive one. Animals, including people, learn faster from pain than from pleasure.

Most people will work harder to avoid losing something they have than they'll work to gain the same thing, creating a strong resistance to change. Hanson writes that our brain is like Velcro for negative experiences and like Teflon for positive ones. That pushes our feelings, expectations, beliefs, and moods in an increasingly negative direction. It makes it harder to be positive, grateful, and giving to others.

But by challenging ourselves to concentrate on positive thinking, we can defy this human built-in negativity bias. We can really highlight our positive experiences and emotions, make a point to concentrate on it, get to know it, enjoy it. We can create a "positive internal reference bank," really highlight it for ourselves, make a point to really enjoy the positive feelings about ourselves, others, and the world around us. In effect, we can re-wire our brains for happiness! This conclusion is firmly grounded in neuroscience, and supported by the discovery that the brain is neuroplastic and can be changed or be rewired.

Rick Hanson's research backs up Saakvine and Pearlman's conclusion that anytime we consciously challenge our negative assumptions and beliefs, we reclaim or create meaning, thus actively transforming vicarious trauma. Creating meaning is on the opposite end of the spectrum from the erosion of beliefs and assumptions trauma professionals face while suffering from vicarious trauma. One may create meaning through challenging oneself to discover importance and substance in everyday life activities. Through mindful awareness, connecting with all aspects of our lives becomes easier, thereby helping trauma professionals to foster gratitude and appreciation for people and things in their lives. Engaging in community-building activities, whether this community is our family, school, workplace, or politically-affiliated group, challenges and offsets the physical, psychological, emotional, and spiritual isolation of vicarious traumatization.

Here are some examples of how can we apply this fascinating scientific stuff in our everyday life. Chances are you remember that supervisor's evaluation that had 30 positive points and one negative. Or that "To Do List" with one incomplete task out of ten. Or that one paper you got a B on in college. The common denominator here is that ONE negative thing, and I bet you remember it much better than all those positive things combined, right?

Like me, you may be your own worst critic. I know that many people I have worked with in the past struggle with same thing. I have found one of the best exercises for fostering that positive internal reference about oneself is to overcome the negative by drowning it out with the positive.

What I do is create a list of "100 Things I Love About Myself.": Then, in times of crisis, when that sneaky self-deprecating thought comes out, ready to strike me at my weak spot, I break out this list to remind myself, that in fact, I am not a loser, but a beautiful, creative, talented, and fascinating child of this Universe!

Yes, it takes effort to write, and double effort to remember to use it against your own negatively biased mind. But with practice, you will enjoy the absence of the inner critic, and instead, will feel the budding presence of self-love and appreciation.

Here are 20 randomly selected items from my "100 Things I Love About Myself" list. Please use it as a baseline or a source of inspiration for your own list. Remember, happiness is a journey, not a destination!

1. I love that I am NOT afraid to take risks.

2. I am adventurous.

3. I am a loving and supportive sister.

4. I am a resilient survivor.

5. I respect and love diversity of any kind, which makes me open-minded and accepting.

6. I am strongly, profoundly committed to my recovery from trauma and everything else I struggle with.

7. I am committed to personal improvement and growth.

8. I am not afraid to be honest with myself and others.

9. I have guts.

10. I have strong drive and passion to make this world a better place.

11. I love my eyes, my hair, my breasts, my butt, my thighs, my legs, my feet.

12. I recognize my strengths.

13. I'm a great swimmer and love water.

14. I am authentic.

15. I am funny.

16. I am a loyal and trustworthy friend.

17. I am very curious and interested.

18. I enjoy bonding and connecting with people.

19. I am a loving mother to my feline babies.

20. I take steps towards achieving my goals and dreams.

I hope you have a very enjoyable self-discovery journey with writing your own list! Don't wait another minute to know and appreciate YOU!

Gratitude

Gratitude is another way to beat the negativity bias and build up your internal positive reference bank. Gratitude supports the sense of fulfillment, appreciation of what we already have. As we know, dissatisfaction with oneself and/or one's life leads to suffering. Cultivating a daily "attitude of gratitude" focuses on the positive in life, thus bringing contentment, and shapes our attitude to life in an increasingly positive direction. Dr. Rick Hanson (rickhanson.net) writes about the healing qualities of gratitude. According to Dr. Hanson, gratitude:

- calms down the stress response, which strengthens our immune system so we can better fight off colds supports the neurochemistry of well-being and protects against depression;

- builds resilience, so we can bounce back faster from difficult life events;

- fosters appreciation of people we care about, thus building "social support" systems which provides additional health benefits in itself; and

- shifts our attention away from resentment, regret, and guilt that are the sources of many health problems.

Gratitude List Exercise:

At the beginning or end of each day consider writing a gratitude list. Write down five to ten items you are grateful for right now: your health, your family, your canine/feline children, your education, your job, sunshine, laugher, clean water, a stocked fridge, gas in your car. Take a few moments and focus on these items, and really feel the sense of thankfulness for being healthy, sober, having love of your favorite people, being able to fulfill your dreams, etc. Recognize the fact that overall, you are incredibly blessed to be alive, safe, and protected. Writing a gratitude list daily is sure way to build new positive pathways in our brain, to create new, positive attitudes, and to become more content and fulfilled.

Be Thankful...

Be thankful that you don't already have
everything you desire.
If you did, what would there be to look forward
to?

Be thankful when you don't know something,
for it gives you the opportunity to learn.

Be thankful for the difficult times.
During those times you grow.

Be thankful for your limitations,
because they give you opportunities for
improvement.

Be thankful for each new challenge,
because it will build your strength and character.

Be thankful for your mistakes.
They will teach you valuable lessons.

Be thankful when you're tired and weary,
because it means you've made a difference.

It's easy to be thankful for the good things.
A life of rich fulfillment comes to those who
are also thankful for the setbacks.

Gratitude can turn a negative into a positive.
Find a way to be thankful for your troubles,
and they can become your blessings.

~Author Unknown

3. Emotional Dimension

Emotional aspects of vicarious trauma prevention follow naturally on the psychological elements, as the two are often intertwined. Here, we start by giving ourselves some emotional breathing room with the practice of self-compassion.

Self-Compassion

Self-compassion is extending compassion to one's self in instances of perceived inadequacy, failure, or general suffering. Dr. Kristin Neff, an Associate Professor in Human Development and Culture, Educational Psychology Department at the University of Texas at Austin and an expert in the field of self-compassion, has defined self-compassion as being composed of three main components: self-kindness, common humanity, and mindfulness. This is what Dr. Neff writes about the three components of self-compassion:

1. *Self-kindness:* Self-compassion is about being gentle and kind to oneself when encountering pain and personal shortcomings, instead of ignoring them or hurting oneself with self-criticism. Self-compassionate people understand that being imperfect, failing, and experiencing life's difficulties is bound to happen, so they tend to be kind with themselves when having painful emotions rather than getting angry at themselves for not being perfect.

2. *Common humanity:* People are often frustrated with themselves and the perceived sense of their singular failure, as if they are the only ones in the whole wide world who ever fail. This is a common and very isolating experience for many. Recognizing that many aspects of ourselves and

the circumstances of our lives are not of our choosing, but instead come from myriad of factors (genetic and/or environmental) that we have little control over may foster empathy for oneself. Self-compassion also involves recognizing that suffering and personal failure is a natural part of the shared human experience.

3. *Mindfulness:* Mindfulness is a non-judgmental, receptive mind-state in which individuals observe their thoughts and feelings as they are, without trying to suppress or deny them. Self-compassionate mindfulness helps balance one's negative emotions so that feelings are neither suppressed nor inflated. Thus, the person is reasonably aware of their emotions without ignoring their feelings or ruminating on them.

What happens when you don't practice self-compassion? Take a look at this blog post from my website (www.olgaphoenix.com) which I wrote after six months of fully supporting myself through my keynotes, trainings, and webinars. I think it clearly shows the lack of self-compassion that I can exercise sometimes, and how it hurts:

"You know what I do every Wednesday for the past 6 months? I agonize in pain and fear, drowning in the sea of inadequacy and self-flagellation. Reason? Oh, it's nothing, just that I have a webinar every Thursday, where I am supposed to be THE EXPERT on various topics, make suggestions, provide real life solutions to people who are experts themselves. I go to my webinar portal and see 30, 40, 50 people registered who are seeking tools and solutions to improve their work environment, be more effective in helping others, and they count on ME to provide it. My FEAR tells me:" Who are you to provide this sort of advice? What makes you think that you are interesting/engaging/knowledgeable/competent? Nobody

will show up tomorrow! Why don't you settle for mediocre and be satisfied with it!"

FEAR, my ever present "False Evidence Appearing Real", taunts me and tells me lies. It draws horrendous pictures of my business's dismal failure, ensuing poverty, and, finally, homelessness, addiction, and death. Intellectually, I understand my FEAR-my life saving defense mechanism which worked for me during my turbulent and violence-ridden childhood and adolescent years. Long, long ago, my FEAR was not false, but very real tool which kept me ALIVE. My FEAR and I, we survived together back then. Now, twenty years later, I still have to remind myself to breathe many times throughout the day, tell myself that I'm an adult and that I'm safe.

The most overwhelmed, incompetent, and fearful I feel is when I am recognized by others through webinar registrations, trainings and keynotes invitations, when people are seeking my expertise, experience, strength, and hope. It's counter-intuitive, but this is the truth.

I am so grateful that I've been blessed with strong, amazing, fantastically talented women friends! They tell me, they live with FEAR too. It's painful manifestations are a little different for each one of us, but feelings of inadequacy and not measuring up are the same. Intellectually, we understand, that FEAR lies, but it hurts, and sometimes, paralyzes, all the same. Last week I asked my auntie if she ever deals with FEAR. She said: "Of course, I do. It's human nature. You only need to prove it to yourself, everyone else already knows how terrific, capable, and intelligent you are. The trick is to have FEAR and to do it ANYWAY."

I think I'll continue telling my girlfriends how I see them: brave, amazing, life changing, survivors, and thrivers. I will accept as THE TRUTH how they see me too. And

I will continue doing advocacy work, despite my FEAR. I will continue doing it ANYWAY!"

Even though I struggle with my perceived failure and fear often, I also try to exercise some self-compassion through mindful awareness as to what is going on with me and my feelings. Sharing my negative experiences with my support group allows me to break the isolation pattern, and confirm that what I'm feeling is a common part of human experience. Mindfulness, awareness, and sharing allow me to be more gentle and kind with myself. I'm happy to report, that now, many moons after I wrote this blog entry, I don't feel FEAR as acutely as I experienced it then: practice, mindfulness, and self-compassion are doing the trick, I think!:)

4. Spiritual Dimension

Nurturing our spiritual side doesn't necessarily mean adhering to any particular religion or philosophy. Instead, it's a way of supporting the most delicate, and profound, parts of our humanity, the spiritual force that brings all the other parts together.

Meditation

There are hundreds of different types of meditation: walking, mindfulness, loving-kindness, visualization to name a few. I personally love all types of guided meditations, and have a CD with guided relaxation meditation with me at all times. Let's look at some ways you can begin a supportive meditation practice.

Relaxation Meditation

Begin by finding a comfortable, relaxed position. Allow your body to begin to relax.

Breathe in ... and out. Take a cleansing breath in ... and breathe out the tension in your body.

Feel relaxation beginning at the bottom of your feet. It might feel like stepping into a warm bathtub ... or it may feel like a tingling sensation ... or simply calm and loose. Allow the relaxation to spread over your feet, and up to your ankles. Feel the relaxation rising above your ankles, flowing up your lower legs ... to your knees ... continuing up to your upper legs.

Allow the relaxation to continue to spread throughout your body, rising now to your hips and pelvic area ... to your stomach and lower back ... to your chest and upper back.

Let your upper arms relax ... your elbows ... lower arms ... and wrists ... feel the relaxation spread to your hands ... relaxing the palms of your hands ... the back of your hands ... each finger and thumb ... your hands feel pleasantly warm, heavy, and relaxed. Allow your shoulders to ease back slightly.

Allow your upper back to relax even further ... let your shoulders relax ... and your neck. Feel the relaxation continue to spread to your chin ... the back of your head ... your mouth ... your cheeks ... nose ... eyes ... Feel your eyelids, heavy and relaxed.

Notice your eyebrows relaxing ... your ears relaxing ... and your forehead ... Your forehead feels cool and relaxed. Let the relaxation spread further to the top of your head.

Your entire body now is relaxed and calm. Feel the relaxation flowing throughout your body, from your head to your feet.

Breathe in ... now hold that breath. And relax your muscles totally, allowing the breath to flow gently out your nose or mouth. Take another deep breath, breathing in relaxation.

And release the breath. Breathe out any remaining tension. Continue to breathe smoothly and slowly as you mentally scan your body, looking for any remaining tension.

If you notice any tension, focus on that area. Direct the relaxation to flow into that area, and then carry the tension away.

Imagine that the air you are breathing can cleanse your body and remove tension. Imagine that each breath in carries relaxation. Picture the tension in your body leaving with each breath out.

Now simply relax, calmly, enjoying the feeling of relaxation for a few moments. (pause)

Now I invite you to return to your usual level of wakefulness and alertness, feel your body and mind becoming more aware of your surroundings.

I will count to three. When I reach three, you will be at your desired level of relaxation or alertness.

1, 2, 3

Healing Meditation

Sitting comfortably or lying down with eyes closed, let's begin by becoming aware of the breath.

Feel the breath as it enters with a cool feeling in your nostrils, in and out....in and out....Fill the lungs with a deep inhale, bringing in energy and light, cleansing and healing.

As you exhale, imagine you body releasing all of negativity, stress, and pain in the air, never to be found again.

Continue like this, breathing in energy and healing light and exhaling negative energy, pain, and stress. In and out...In and out...

Become aware of the healing light touching every cell in your body, bringing warmth and joy, starting with the crown of your head.

Feel it starting to travel down into your body from the top of your head, slowly going down into your face and neck, traveling down into the shoulders, all the way down into the arms, down to the fingers.

Feel the healing energy and light going down into your chest, all the way down to your hips. Feel it continue traveling down your legs all the way down to your toes.

Your whole body is now filled with healing light and energy. Allow that healing energy to completely fill any physical area that needs healing energy.

Feel it warming, healing and expanding through the area. Allow the healing light to bring peace and healing to every organ, tissue, and emotion in your body and mind.

Feel healing energy revitalizing and nurturing your body and mind.

Stay with this deep, relaxing, peaceful feeling of blissful healing and wellness.

When you are ready, feel your body and mind becoming more aware of your surroundings, feeling wakeful and alert.

I will count to three. When I reach three, you will return to the room, relaxed, rejuvenated, and healed.

1, 2, 3

5. Personal Dimension

Fostering rich personal life is extremely important. It may seem selfish to focus on yourself when you know how much suffering others are going through, but it's necessary for you and for those you help.

Affirmations

An affirmation is a positive statement of what you want in your life, expressed in the present tense. Affirmations are the tools for creating something you want, by "tricking" your mind to believe the stated concept while beating the negativity bias and building up your internal positive reference bank.

Example: "I'm remarkable and cherished; I can and I do."

Healing Affirmation

My mind, my body, and my soul are free, healed, and whole.

I welcome unconditional love, healing, happiness, and peace to enter my being and live here.

I commit to a life abundant in unconditional love, healing, happiness, and peace to be with me always.

It is a way of life for me now.

Affirmation About Relationships

I am happy, healthy, balanced, and whole.

I have wonderful, healthy, and balanced relationships in all areas of my life.

I am loved, respected, and cherished by my family, friends, and intimate partner,

and I love, respect, and cherish them in return.

Love for my family, friends, and intimate partner is easy, healthy, and fulfilling.

Affirmation About Intimate Relationship

I love my partner, who is my equal,

and loving them is effortless, satisfying, and a gift.

We love each other unconditionally,

and it feels supportive, gentle, healthy, and whole.

Our relationship is healthy, balanced, and strong.

Loving each other is easy, fulfilling, and a gift.

Thank you, Universe, for my ability to give and receive love.

Here is one about fulfilling one's goals and dreams. This is the real life affirmation I said out loud every morning for a few months to make this book happen! (don't get me wrong, I had to write it! But affirming it daily gave me the strength and willingness to do it, I'm pretty sure of it!:).

Affirmation About This Book

Thank you, Universe, for the success of my book.

Thank you for its smooth writing, production, and publication process,

And best-selling title! :D

Thank you for giving me direction and knowledge as to who to work with on my book.

Thank you for providing me with all financial support I need to make the book happen.

Thank you for my ability to help so much more people through my book.

There can be no delay, impediment, or obstruction to the realization of my heart's desire.

The Power of the Universe is now moving on my behalf!

P.S. If you are reading this book in print or in

ebook-see, this affirmation worked!:D

A friend sent this powerful affirmation to me. Originally, it was supposed to be "101 Ways to Praise Your Child", Author Unknown-you can find posters like this online and at any teacher's store. I promptly adopted it into "101 Ways to Praise Yourself". For all the grown victim advocates who get to parent themselves! Here's an Empowerment Affirmation you can look at every day:

101 WAYS TO PRAISE YOURSELF☺

WOW • WAY TO GO • SUPER • YOU'RE SPECIAL • OUTSTANDING • EXCELLENT •GREAT• GOOD • NEAT • WELL DONE • REMARKABLE • I KNEW YOU COULD DO IT •I'M PROUD OF YOU • FANTASTIC • SUPER STAR • NICE WORK • LOOKING GOOD • YOU'RE ON TOP OF IT • BEAUTIFUL • NOW YOU'RE FLYING • YOU'RE CATCHING ON • NOW YOU'VE GOT IT • YOU'RE INCREDIBLE • BRAVO • YOU'RE FANTASTIC • HURRAY FOR YOU • YOU'RE ON TARGET • YOU'RE ON YOUR WAY • HOW NICE • HOW SMART • GOOD JOB • THAT'S INCREDIBLE • HOT DOG • DYNAMITE • YOU'RE BEAUTIFUL • YOU'RE UNIQUE • NOTHING CAN STOP YOU NOW • GOOD FOR YOU • I LIKE YOU YOU'RE A WINNER • REMARKABLE JOB • BEAUTIFUL WORK • SPECTACULAR • YOU'RE SPECTACULAR • YOU'RE DARLING • YOU'RE PRECIOUS • GREAT DISCOVERY • YOU'VE DISCOVERED THE SECRET • YOU FIGURED IT OUT • FANTASTIC JOB • BINGO • MAGNIFICENT • MARVELOUS • TERRIFIC • YOU'RE IMPORTANT• PHENOMENAL • YOU'RE SENSATIONAL • SUPER WORK • CREATIVE JOB • SUPER JOB• FANTASTIC JOB • EXCEPTIONAL PERFORMANCE • YOU'RE A REAL TROOPER • YOU ARE RESPONSIBLE • YOU ARE EXCITING • YOU LEARNED IT RIGHT • WHAT AN IMAGINATION •WHAT A GOOD LISTENER • YOU ARE FUN • YOU'RE GROWING UP • YOU TRIED HARD • YOU CARE • BEAUTIFUL SHARING • OUTSTANDING PERFORMANCE • YOU'RE A GOOD FRIEND • I TRUST YOU • YOU'RE IMPORTANT • YOU MEAN A LOT TO ME • YOU MAKE ME HAPPY • YOU BELONG • YOU'VE GOT A FRIEND • YOU MAKE ME LAUGH • YOU BRIGHTEN MY DAY • I RESPECT YOU • YOU MEAN THE WORLD TO ME • YOU'RE A JOY • YOU'RE A TREASURE • YOU'RE WONDERFUL • YOU'RE PERFECT • I LOVE YOU!

Bringing it All Together

One way to consolidate all of the work you do on the various dimensions is to put it down on paper. Journals are good, but visual reminders have their own special power. One helpful exercise is the vision board.

Creating Meaning and a Full Life with Vision Board

A Vision Board is a collection of images, words and colors which reflect your visions and desires for your life. It is a tool which allows you to become clear on what you really want. Becoming clear on what you want is the key to manifesting your vision. Brainstorm about what you'd like your life to be like, and put your dreams as a collage on a large sheet of paper. Put it in a prominent place in your home to remind yourself daily about your goals and dreams.

Here is an example of one of my Vision Boards (Figure 6). You'll notice it doesn't have to be all serious stuff. You can see where my priorities lie: a large portion of the space is dedicated to Moorea, Tahiti, my fantasy island where I shall go sooner than later! Next comes completing my Ph.D. and writing tons of books, which most definitely will hold best-selling titles. The third place is dedicated to healthy eating habits, workout routines, and maintaining perpetual serenity in all areas of life. It's your Vision Board, be bold, reach for the stars, imagine the life you want to live!

Figure 6. Olga's Vision Board graphic.

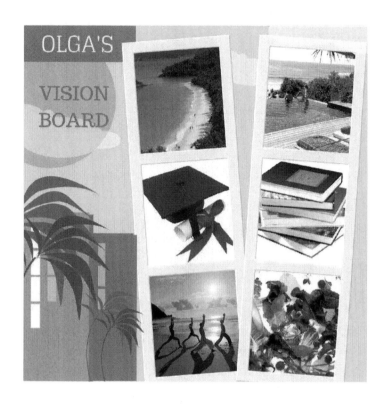

10 Steps Closer to Your Dreams through a Vision Board

Create a collection of images, words and colors which reflect your visions and desires for your life. This is a tool which allows you to become clear on what you really want. Becoming clear on what you want is the key to manifesting your vision.

Step One:

Gather magazines and catalogues.

Step Two:

Go through the magazines and catalogues and pull out images, words and phrases that speak to you or evoke feelings.

Step Three:

Cut out these images and words.

Step Four:

Place your words and images on a large board in

a way that feels right to you.

Step Five:

Paste the images on the board.

Step Six:

Review your Board and ask yourself what do you need to do in order to accomplish your dreams.

Step Seven:

Create a reasonable and achievable plan of action.

Step Eight:

Find support for changing your life. Share your dream board with a friend.

Step Nine:

Create a "buddy system of accountability" with a friend in order to stay on track.

Step Ten:

Place the board somewhere you'll see it every day. Accomplish your visions, ONE STEP at a TIME!

6. Professional Dimension

As victim advocates, we tend to hang out in this dimension quite a lot, and sometimes way too much. For some of us, the main goal is to establish boundaries between professional and other dimensions in our life. For others, it maybe the matter of taking lunch outside, away from the computer screen (with grant reports on it). And quite possibly, most of us could benefit from an extra dose of attitude of gratitude and mindful appreciation at the office. Here are some suggestions.

"Leaving Work At Work" Rituals

Hundreds of advocates told me that victims comes home with us, in our thoughts, in our dreams. I like to make a not-so-funny joke that sometimes victims come home with us, sit at our dinner table, and even as we try to catch a little sleep, their faces, and their eyes stare from the pillow right next to us! Sometimes the situation is really acute, to the point of nightmares or insomnia, and sometimes it's just passing but nagging thoughts "Is she ok? Did I help her enough? Did I do all I could do in the situation?" (Please consider seeing a counselor if you are concerned about your wellbeing. Talking the situation out with a professional greatly reduces the power of negative thoughts, emotions, and feelings. Plus, they always have a great advice on how to deal with a situation-win/win overall!).

I think it's really really important for all of us to develop our own trusted 'leaving work at work rituals"-practices that give cues to our body and mind that work is over and it's time to play and relax. This about the following questions: Is there anything that you do that helps you to leave work at work? Do you have any ritual that you follow at the end of your workday?

Rituals that advocates told me about:

- Watering plants at work before going home
- Studying foreign language on the way home
- Singing with favorite band on the way home
- Taking 15-60 min to yourself before engaging with family
- Taking a shower right after work and imagining that work stress goes right down the drain
- Taking all work clothes off as a symbol of taking off all of your stresses
- Playing with pets for a while when arriving home
- Gardening right after work
- Burning sage at home after work to purify your spirit
- For the next week, experiment with a specific ritual, reflecting on how it affects you.

Examples of Professional Dimension Activities

Sometimes looking at the big picture is helpful, and at other times, you simply want a bag of tools to reach into to help you get through the day. Here are some simple and practical ideas to brighten up your work day:

- Balance your caseload so that no one day or part of a day is "too much" (ex.: don't cram tasks you dislike in one day).

- "Mix and Match" your favorite projects with not so favorite ones all throughout the day.

- Get regular supervision or consultation (ex.: trust and team cohesiveness can be developed through reflective supervision practices).

- Remember to plan ahead and take your personal, vacation, sick, and mental health days.

- Take a break during the workday and leave the office (ex.: out for lunch, even if it means tuna sandwich from home on the bench by your office building).

- Honor those who have gone before you by agreeing to adhere to sustainable and reasonable work schedule. This means 9-5 and lots of play time outside of work!

- Incorporate gratitude into your work day (ex.: think of 1 thing you are grateful for in the beginning and the end of your workday, right it down in your work gratitude journal-for future reverences, when you need a "pick-me-up").

- Think about people in your life you are grateful for and tell them about it (ex.:

write a thank you card to a coworker who taught you something recently).

- Express your gratitude and compliment your coworkers often.

- Accept compliments graciously, and allow yourself to feel "pretty, smart, stylish, etc" (ex.: just say "thank you" and take a moment to appreciate yourself)

- Develop a vicarious trauma prevention support group at work (ex.: the only rule being that you have to come up with vicarious trauma prevention solutions, rather than discussing vicarious trauma problems).

- Develop a non-trauma area of professional interest (ex.: try your skill in writing steamy romance novels on the side or take a drawing class).

- Write down your own strategies and practice them often.

Your Professional Vicarious Trauma Prevention Exercise

Understanding yourself is the first step toward making positive, self-affirming choices. Here are some prompts to get you started. You may want to journal your answers, or share your thoughts with a friend, counselor, or a trusted colleague.

1.Why did you choose trauma-related work?

2.How do you sustain and nurture yourself daily/weekly/monthly/yearly?

3.Provided that vicarious trauma prevention is 2-fold, what are your

a. "self-care/escape" activities?

b. "creating meaning in your life" activities?

4. Now that you know VT prevention tools, how will you live your life differently, in all six dimensions of it?

5. Do you still think this is the right career path for you?

CHAPTER 4:

ORGANIZATIONAL CULTURE OF VICARIOUS TRAUMA PREVENTION AND SUSTAINABILITY

Research by John Fawcett (2003; 2011) shows that the single most important factor that negatively impacts health and well-being in organizational contexts is the organization itself: how the agency works, how leadership relates to staff, what kind of human resource support systems are present, whether teams are cohesive, and whether the context and culture of the organization is supportive of growth and development. Employment conditions have significant influence on the health and well-being of staff.

Fawcett asserts that organizational leadership, including members of the Board of Directors, have a primary ethical responsibility for creating environments for staff that promote health and support individual vicarious trauma prevention. Individual vicarious trauma prevention efforts work, but in organizations where people are denied the opportunity to make use of these skills and knowledge, individual health suffers. Organizations have significant capacity, and responsibility, to create supportive work environments. These efforts not only protect employees from the negative impact of vicarious trauma, but also enhance the chances staff members will actually thrive in challenging environments.

Such changes can be very difficult, because the organization itself might be entrenched in trauma. Various authors within the trauma field have written about the fundamental processes of post-traumatic reactivity and the negative effects of trauma on an organization as a whole. For example, Sandra Bloom, founder of the Sanctuary Model, addresses how trauma can contaminate an organization's processes and policies; she underscores how organizations meant to serve traumatized populations can themselves become neglectful and hurtful to their staff and clients. Bloom proposes a solution: creating trauma-informed processes and policies that support the wellbeing and health of the staff and the people they serve.

Of course, it is sometimes difficult to even take the first steps toward change within an organization. It's often a challenge to persuade leaders that there is a significant return on investment in allowing and encouraging staff to "take time away from work" to enter these practices. You may have to convince them that a healthy workforce is worth the investment.

Another roadblock you may face when working with leaders of trauma organizations is that they may allow staff to practice vicarious trauma prevention, but not participate themselves. Staff members know when their supervisors are only giving lip service to a new policy or procedure. Vicarious trauma prevention practices are more likely to be sustained over time where leadership, including board members, are actively and personally engaged in such vicarious trauma prevention practices themselves, preferably in the same context as other staff.

Implementing these vicarious trauma prevention practices can be challenging, and unfortunately, the changes are not likely to be sustainable in the face of such a split between management and staff. Staff might perceive themselves as being less competent than managers who feel they don't need this extra help, or they may become convinced that management wants them to practice vicarious trauma prevention because staff is doing something wrong or not effectively. Overall, there's a sense that managers are not at all invested in the staff's well-being.

The message needs to come from the top if lasting changes are to be made. Ultimately, accountability—along with the ethical responsibility for fostering organizational cultures of vicarious trauma prevention, self-care, wellness, and sustainability—rests in the hands of organizational leadership. With strong organizational leadership, the staff can then take on a stronger role in maintaining a healthy workplace for all.

"How Healthy is Your Organization" Exercise

- How does the agency work?
- How does leadership relate to staff?
- What kind of human resource support systems are present?
- How cohesive are teams?
- Is the context and culture of the organization supportive of growth and development?
- Is vicarious trauma prevention encouraged? If so, how?
- Is vicarious trauma prevention practiced by teams and leadership? If so, how?

If you see some work to be done based on your answers, remember, it is not a problem, but rather a fantastic opportunity for growth. It's about turning problems into possibilities. It is about consciously choosing to see what can be done, rather than staying with how you dislike the situation. It is committing to discovering fascinating possibilities and growing individually and as an organization. And being effective. And being well.

Vicarious Trauma Prevention Practices and Organizational Sustainability

Leadership, including Boards of Directors, has primary ethical responsibility for creating environments which promote and support organizational and individual vicarious trauma prevention. While personal efforts are important, individual health can still be compromised in contexts where people are denied the opportunity to make use of these skills and knowledge. The most effective way to address and prevent vicarious trauma is through sound organizational processes. Here are some examples of what leadership could do to promote wellness of an organization overall:

- provide sufficient training for every member of your team on vicarious trauma, it's symptoms, effects, and tools to address and prevent it.

- assure your staff that vicarious trauma symptoms are a completely normal reaction to trauma work and encourage them to seek help.

- establish organizational systems of care for victim advocates who disclose or present with vicarious trauma symptoms.

- provide adequate training in trauma-specific and trauma-informed outreach, intake, and service delivery strategies, to increase victim advocates' sense of effectiveness in helping clients and reduces the sense of demoralization brought on by trauma work.

- establish a diverse caseload of clients in order to limit the traumatic exposure of any one worker.

- create work environments which facilitate staff bonding and emotional support of each other, as this limits emotional fatigue and depersonalization, and creates a greater sense of personal accomplishment (e.g.: a vicarious trauma prevention support group).

- institute regular relationally based clinical supervision to normalize victim advocates' feelings and experiences and provide support and tools to address and prevent vicarious trauma.

- provide safe and comfortable space for victim advocates to engage in their personal vicarious trauma prevention activities during the work day (e.g.: therapy, 12 step meetings, meditation, long lunch with support group).

- nurture a culture of shared power in making organizational decisions, empower a sense of autonomy in victim advocates, as trust, empowerment, and self-efficacy are the antidotes to a sense of powerlessness associated with vicarious trauma.

- as an organization, start taking steps towards improving your organizational health and practices.

CONCLUSION

The research collected in the past twenty years is consistent: many trauma professionals, specifically domestic/sexual violence advocates, are at risk for vicarious traumatization and compassion fatigue. The research identifies major risk factors for secondary traumatic stress and vicarious trauma, such as: being less experienced, having a personal trauma history, and having a

127

greater exposure to traumatized individuals such as those with a heavier caseload of survivors.

However, vicarious trauma is preventable. Through employing sustainable and preventive self-care, nurturing, and escape activities, trauma professionals can mitigate the stress of vicarious trauma. Through the processes of creating meaning, challenging negative beliefs and assumptions, and participating in community-building activities, trauma professionals can transform the despair, demoralization, and loss of hope produced by vicarious traumatization.

Although prevention of vicarious trauma on a personal level is very useful, unhealthy organizational climates may reduce the positive effects of personal self-care dramatically. The effectiveness of organizational policies of vicarious trauma prevention and sustainability often rests in the hands of leadership. Management team members of trauma organizations are ethically responsible for implementing, empowering, and practicing the organizational culture of vicarious trauma prevention and wellness in order to not only provide the most beneficial services to trauma survivors, but to keep sustainable, empowering, and healthy work environments for their staff.

Having read this book, you now have some tools to begin preventing and treating vicarious trauma in your own life, as well as bringing the problem and its solutions to the attention of management and institutions as a whole. With healthier workforces, agencies that help trauma victims will ultimately be more successful in their core goal: helping more people more effectively.

MY PERSONAL NOTE TO YOU

On my amazing, meandering journey to a life free of vicarious trauma, I have encountered many teachers. They came in many forms: an insightful therapist, a burned out colleague, a kind spiritual teacher, the raw pain of untreated trauma, a thousand and one books read on the topics of world's healing spiritual practices, deep depression, and the intense joy of witnessing victims of violence recover.

What I learned is that the common threads in any journey to balance and wellness are self-awareness, self-love, self-compassion, self-forgiveness, moderation, and development of a positive personal identity. This means learning to think of ourselves outside of our role as a victim advocate, and being completely okay with just "I AM." That's a complete sentence: I AM. Period.

Now, having read this book, I hope that you are closer to embracing this new perspective: "I AM, and I deserve my place on this planet, and I have a right to be well, happy, and live a life free of vicarious trauma."

REFERENCES

Abendroth, M. & Flannery, J.(2006). Predicting the risk of compassion fatigue: A study of hospice nurses. *Journal of Hospice and Palliative Nursing*, 8(6), 346-356.

Adams, R. E., Boscarino, J. A., & Figley, C. R. (2006). *Compassion fatigue and psychological distress among social workers: A validation study. American Journal of Orthopsychiatry, 76(1), 103-108.*

Albers, S. (2009). *50 Ways to Soothe Yourself Without Food.* Oakland, Calif.: New Harbinger Publications.

Bell, H., Kulkarni, S. & Dalton, L. (2003). Organizational prevention of vicarious trauma. *Families in Society*, 84(4), 463-470.

Bloom, S. & Farragher, B. (2013). *Restoring Sanctuary: A New Operating System for Trauma-Informed Systems of Care.* Oxford University Press.

Bober, T. & Regehr, C. (2006). Strategies for reducing secondary or vicarious trauma: Do they work? *Brief Treatment and Crisis Intervention, 6*, 1–9.

Bride, B. E. (2007). Prevalence of secondary traumatic stress among social workers. *Social Work*, 52(1), 63–70.

Conrad, D., & Kellar-Guenther, Y. (2006). Compassion fatigue, burnout, and compassion satisfaction among Colorado child protection workers. *Child Abuse and Neglect*, 30(10), 1071-1080.

Cornille, T. A., & Meyers, T. W. (1999). Secondary traumatic stress among child protective service workers: Prevalence, severity and predictive factors. *Traumatology*, 5(1), 15-31.

Curtis, L. (2010). Case backload postponing deportations proceedings increases 26 percent, but immigration judges swamped. *Las Vegan Review Journal*, May 30.

Decker, S., & Naugle, A. (2008). DBT for Sexual Abuse Survivors: Current Status and Future Directions. *Journal of Behavior Analysis of Offender and Victim: Treatment and Prevention*, 1(4): 52–69.

Dernoot Lypsky, L. (2009). *Trauma Stewardship: An Everyday Gide to Caring for Self while Caring for Others.* Berrett-Koehler Publishers, San Francisco, CA.

Fawcett, J. (2003). Assessing front-line staff for stress, trauma, and social support: Theory, practice, and implications, In *Stress and trauma handbook: Strategies for flourishing in demanding environments*. Monrovia, CA: World Vision International.

Fawcett, J. (2011).Organizational and Cultural Factors that Promote Coping: With Reference to Haiti and Christchurch, *New Zealand Journal of Psychology*, no. 4 (Vol. 40).

Figley, C. (1995). *Compassion Fatigue: Coping With Secondary Traumatic Stress Disorder In Those Who Treat The Traumatized*. Routledge Psychosocial Stress Series.

Figley, C. (1995). Compassion fatigue as secondary traumatic stress disorder: An overview. In C. R. Figley (Ed.), *Compassion fatigue: Coping with secondary traumatic stress disorder in those who treat the traumatized*. New York: Brunner/Mazel.

Hanson, R. (2011). *Just One Thing: Developing a Buddha Brain One Simple Practice at a Time*. Oakland, Calif.: New Harbinger Publications.

Hawkins, H.C. (2001). Police officer burnout: A partial replication of Maslach's burnout inventory. *Police Quarterly*, 4(3), 343-360.

Janssen, M. (2009). *Pleasure Healing: Mindful Practices & Sacred Spa Rituals for Self-Nurturing.* New Harbinger Publications, Inc.

Linehan, M. (1993). *Skills Training Manual for Treating Borderline Personality Disorder.* The Guilford Press; 1st edition.

Lobel, J. (1997). The vicarious effects of treating female rape survivors: The therapist's

perspective. (Doctoral Dissertation, University of Pennsylvania, 1997). Dissertation Abstracts

International: Section B: *The Sciences and Engineering,* Vol 57(11-B), May 1997. pp. 7230.

Mathieu, F. (2012). *The Compassion Fatigue Workbook.* Routledge, NY.

Neff, K.D. The development and validation of a scale to measure self-compassion. *Self and Identity,* **2**(3): 223–250.

Newell, J. M. & MacNeil, G. A. (2010). Professional burnout, vicarious trauma, secondary traumatic stress, and compassion fatigue: A review of theoretical terms, risk factors, andpreventive methods for clinicians and researchers. *Best Practices in Mental Health: An International Journal, 6,* 57-68.

Perez, L. M., Jones, J., Englert, D. R., & Sachau, D. (2010). Secondary traumatic stress and burnout among law enforcement investigators exposed to disturbing media images. *Journal of Police and Criminal Psychology,* 25(2), 113-124.

Perron, B., & Hiltz, B. (2006). Burnout and secondary trauma among forensic interviewers of abused children. *Child and Adolescent Social Work Journal,* 23(2), 216-234.

Saakvitne, K. & Pearlman, L. (1996). *Transforming the Pain: A Workbook on Vicarious Traumatization.* Norton Publishing, NY.

Stamm, B.H. (2010). *The Concise ProQol Manual.*2nd Edition. Pocatello, ID:ProQol.org; 2010.

Stamm, B.H. (2012). *The ProQOL (Professional Quality of Life Scale: Compassion Satisfaction and Compassion Fatigue).* Retrieved: May 1, 2014 from proqol.org.

ABOUT THE AUTHOR

Olga Phoenix is a national speaker, trainer, and an advocate. She is a founder and president of Olga Phoenix Project: Healing for Social Change, an organization dedicated to foster vicarious trauma prevention among trauma professionals. She is a Department of Justice Office for Victims of Crime Training and Technical Assistance Center expert consultant and trainer on vicarious trauma prevention; and a member of training and mentoring team at the National Partnership to End Interpersonal Violence. Olga Phoenix graduated with a Masters of Public Administration and Nonprofit Management from the University of South Florida, Masters of Arts in Women's Studies from Florida Atlantic University, and is currently a Doctorate Candidate at the California Institute of Integral Studies. She lives in San Francisco, CA with her two feline children.

Made in the USA
Middletown, DE
26 July 2017